Living With Herpes

A Comprehensive Guide to Understanding and Treating Herpes

Dr. Sarah White

TABLE OF CONTENT

Introduction

Welcome to "Living With Herpes" : A Comprehensive Guide to Understanding and Treating Herpes." In this book, we embark on a journey through the intricate landscape of herpes, providing a thorough exploration of its types, historical context, and the profound impact it has on individuals. The initial chapter acts as a compass, encapsulating essential information on herpes, setting the stage for a deeper dive into effective treatment strategies.

As we progress, the focus shifts towards empowering readers with practical insights and targeted solutions. Our goal is not only to inform but to equip individuals with the knowledge they need to navigate the challenges posed by herpes. From antiviral medications to personalized remedies for specific types of herpes, each chapter unveils a spectrum of approaches. Emphasizing prevention, emotional support, and dispelling societal stigma, "Herpes Unveiled" is not just a book; it's a companion in the journey toward understanding, treating, and overcoming the complexities of living with herpes.

Comprehensive Overview of Herpes

Definition and Types

Herpes, a viral infection caused by the herpes simplex virus (HSV) and the varicella-zoster virus (VZV), manifests in various forms, each presenting unique challenges. The two primary types of herpes simplex viruses are HSV-1 and HSV-2.

1. Herpes Simplex Virus Type 1 (HSV-1):
   - Oral Herpes: Commonly associated with cold sores or fever blisters, HSV-1 typically affects the mouth and facial areas.
   - Transmission: Spread through oral-to-oral contact, often during childhood through nonsexual interactions.

2. Herpes Simplex Virus Type 2 (HSV-2):
   - Genital Herpes: Primarily affects the genital and anal regions, causing painful sores and ulcers.
   - Transmission: Mainly through sexual contact, HSV-2 is a leading cause of genital herpes.

3. Varicella-Zoster Virus (VZV):
   - Chickenpox: VZV causes chickenpox, characterized by itchy skin rashes and flu-like symptoms.
   - Shingles: After chickenpox, the virus may reactivate, leading to shingles, a painful rash typically affecting one side of the body.

Understanding these types is crucial for diagnosis and effective management. HSV infections are chronic, with the virus residing in nerve cells, periodically causing outbreaks. VZV, on the other hand, exhibits a dormant phase but may reactivate, emphasizing the importance of comprehensive knowledge for individuals and healthcare providers alike.

Historical Context

The historical context of herpes is a narrative that spans centuries, reflecting the evolving understanding and societal perceptions of this viral infection.

1. Ancient Times:

- References to symptoms resembling herpes date back to ancient civilizations, with descriptions in texts from Greece, Rome, and Egypt.
- Limited medical knowledge often led to the association of herpes with supernatural causes or divine punishment.

2. Middle Ages:
- Lack of medical advancements perpetuated misconceptions and stigmatization of individuals with visible symptoms, contributing to societal fears.

3. Renaissance and Early Modern Period:
- Advancements in medical science during the Renaissance led to a more systematic exploration of diseases, but herpes remained poorly understood.
- Historical records indicate outbreaks of what may have been herpes, but clear differentiation between HSV-1 and HSV-2 was not established.

4. 20th Century:
- Breakthroughs in virology and medical technology facilitated the identification of herpes viruses.

- The 1960s marked the isolation of HSV-1 and HSV-2, distinguishing between oral and genital herpes.
- The introduction of antiviral medications in the late 20th century provided a means for symptom management.

5. Recent Advances:
- Ongoing research aims to unravel the complex nature of herpes, exploring antiviral resistance, vaccines, and novel treatment modalities.
- Societal attitudes have evolved with increased awareness and education, challenging the historical stigma associated with herpes.

Understanding the historical context of herpes underscores the progress made in unraveling its mysteries, dispelling myths, and fostering a more compassionate and informed approach to this prevalent viral infection. The journey from ancient misconceptions to contemporary medical insights highlights the importance of ongoing research and awareness in shaping our understanding of herpes.

Chapter 1

Understanding Herpes

In this foundational chapter, we embark on a comprehensive exploration of herpes, delving into its intricate facets to equip readers with a nuanced understanding. From the causes and modes of transmission to the subtle nuances of symptoms and their impact on health, this chapter lays the groundwork for a deeper dive into the world of herpes. By unraveling the mysteries surrounding this viral infection, we pave the way for informed discussions on treatment strategies, prevention, and the emotional landscape of living with herpes. Join us on a journey of knowledge, as we navigate the complexities of herpes, providing essential insights that empower individuals to face the challenges posed by this prevalent and often misunderstood condition.

Causes, Transmission, and Symptoms

Causes:

Herpes is caused by the herpes simplex virus (HSV) and the varicella-zoster virus (VZV). HSV has two primary types, HSV-1 and HSV-2, which are responsible for oral and genital herpes, respectively. VZV causes chickenpox and can later reemerge as shingles.

Transmission:
1. HSV-1 Transmission:
   - Oral-to-Oral: Commonly transmitted through direct contact with oral secretions, such as kissing or sharing utensils.
   - Nonsexual Contact: Childhood transmission often occurs through nonsexual interactions.

2. HSV-2 Transmission:
   - Sexual Contact: Mainly transmitted through sexual activities involving genital, anal, or oral regions.
   - Vertical Transmission: Can be transmitted from an infected mother to her newborn during childbirth

3. VZV Transmission:
   - Airborne and Direct Contact: Chickenpox spreads through respiratory droplets or direct contact with the rash.
   - Reactivation: Shingles can be transmitted through direct contact with the rash during its active phase.

Symptoms:

1. HSV-1 Symptoms:
   - Cold Sores: Painful, fluid-filled blisters on or around the lips.
   - Fever and Fatigue: Accompanied by flu-like symptoms during initial outbreaks

2. HSV-2 Symptoms:
   - Genital Sores: Painful ulcers on the genital or anal regions.
   - Flu-like Symptoms: Fever, headache, and muscle aches during primary outbreaks.

3. VZV Symptoms:
   - Chickenpox: Itchy rash, fever, and flu-like symptoms.

- Shingles: Painful rash with blisters, often localized to one side of the body.

Understanding the causes, modes of transmission, and diverse symptoms associated with these herpes viruses is pivotal for accurate diagnosis, effective management, and preventive measures. The intricate interplay of these elements contributes to the complex nature of herpes infections, emphasizing the need for comprehensive knowledge in both medical and public health contexts.

Diagnosis and Impact on Health

Diagnosis:

1. Clinical Evaluation:
   - Healthcare professionals often diagnose herpes based on a visual examination of symptoms such as sores or blisters.
   - Medical history, including sexual and medical history, is considered in the diagnostic process.

2. Laboratory Tests:
   - Viral Culture: Collecting a sample from a sore to culture and identify the virus.

- Polymerase Chain Reaction (PCR) Test: Detects viral DNA in blood, tissue, or cerebrospinal fluid.
- Blood Tests: Serologic tests can detect antibodies to HSV, indicating a previous or current infection.

3. Direct Testing:
- Direct Fluorescent Antibody (DFA) Test: Identifies viral antigens in cells.
- Tzanck Smear: Microscopic examination of cells from a blister to detect herpes infection.

Impact on Health:

1. Physical Health:
- Acute Symptoms: Herpes outbreaks can cause pain, itching, and flu-like symptoms.
- Complications: In severe cases, complications such as meningitis or encephalitis can occur.

2. Recurrent Outbreaks:
- Frequency and Severity: Outbreaks vary, with some individuals experiencing frequent and severe episodes, while others have milder or infrequent symptoms.
- Triggers: Factors like stress, illness, or weakened immune function can trigger outbreaks.

3. Psychological and Emotional Impact:
   - Stigma and Emotional Distress: The social stigma associated with herpes can lead to emotional distress and negatively impact mental health.
   - Quality of Life: Individuals may face challenges in relationships, intimacy, and overall quality of life.

4. Prevention of Transmission:
   - Safe Practices: Proper condom use and avoiding sexual activity during outbreaks can reduce the risk of transmission.
   - Antiviral Medications: Medications can help manage symptoms and reduce the risk of transmission.

Understanding the diagnostic methods and the multifaceted impact of herpes on physical and mental health is crucial for individuals, healthcare providers, and the broader community. It forms the basis for developing effective treatment strategies, offering support, and dispelling misconceptions surrounding this common viral infection.

Chapter 2

Treatment Approaches

In this crucial chapter, we explore the dynamic landscape of treating herpes infections, offering a comprehensive guide to diverse strategies aimed at managing symptoms, reducing outbreaks, and enhancing overall well-being. From the general principles guiding antiviral medications and lifestyle modifications to personalized approaches for each type of herpes, this chapter equips readers with practical tools for navigating the complexities of treatment. We delve into the specifics of HSV-1 and HSV-2, addressing both oral and genital herpes, and shed light on targeted therapies for the varicella-zoster virus. With a focus on prevention, risk reduction, and the emotional dimensions of living with herpes, our exploration aims to empower individuals with the knowledge needed to make informed decisions about their health and forge a path toward a balanced and fulfilling life.

General Principles

Antiviral Medications

Antiviral medications play a central role in managing and suppressing herpes infections. These medications aim to reduce the severity and duration of symptoms, alleviate discomfort, and lower the risk of transmission. Here, we explore the key antiviral medications used in the treatment of herpes:

1. Acyclovir:
   - Mechanism of Action: Inhibits viral DNA replication.
   - Forms: Available in oral, topical, and intravenous formulations.
   - Applications: Commonly used for both HSV and VZV infections.

2. Valacyclovir:
   - Prodrug of Acyclovir: Converts to acyclovir in the body, enhancing bioavailability.
   - Convenience: Often preferred due to less frequent dosing compared to acyclovir.
   - Effectiveness: Demonstrates efficacy in managing both oral and genital herpes.

3. Famciclovir:
   - Prodrug of Penciclovir: Converts to penciclovir, inhibiting viral DNA replication.
   - Application: Effective against both HSV and VZV.
   - Dosage: Administered as a convenient, twice-daily oral medication.

4. Penciclovir:
   - Topical Application: Available as a cream for treating recurrent oral herpes (cold sores).
   - Mechanism of Action: Inhibits viral DNA replication.

5. Letermovir:
   - Prevention of Cytomegalovirus (CMV): Used in specific cases, such as transplant recipients at risk for CMV infection.
   - Mechanism: Targets the CMV terminase complex, preventing viral replication.

Considerations:

- Initiation of Treatment: Early initiation of antiviral treatment during the prodromal phase or at the onset of symptoms enhances effectiveness.

- Suppressive Therapy: For individuals with frequent outbreaks, a continuous suppressive therapy approach may be recommended to reduce the frequency and severity of recurrences.

- Pregnancy and Breastfeeding: The choice of antiviral medication during pregnancy requires careful consideration, balancing the benefits of treatment with potential risks.

Understanding the spectrum of antiviral medications empowers individuals and healthcare providers to make informed decisions tailored to specific herpes infections. While these medications offer effective symptom management, ongoing research seeks to advance treatment options and further enhance the quality of life for those affected by herpes.

Chapter 3

Natural Remedies for Herpes treatment

Welcome to a transformative journey exploring the realm of natural remedies for managing herpes. In this chapter, we navigate beyond conventional treatments, delving into the synergistic potential of lifestyle adjustments and herbal interventions. By intertwining the wisdom of nature with evidence-based practices, we aim to empower individuals seeking holistic approaches to herpes management.

Beginning with lifestyle and dietary considerations, we unravel the impact of nutrition, hydration, and stress management on immune health. Our exploration extends to herbal supplements like Echinacea, Lemon Balm, and Licorice Root, dissecting their antiviral properties and safe application methods. Topical remedies, including

Aloe Vera, Coconut Oil, and Tea Tree Oil, take center stage for soothing relief.

Diving into the microbial realm, we uncover the role of probiotics and immune-supportive supplements. Cautionary notes guide readers on consultation with healthcare professionals, potential interactions, and the importance of monitoring for allergic reactions.

As we conclude, this chapter serves as a compass, guiding readers to seamlessly integrate natural remedies into their daily routines, fostering not only herpes management but a holistic approach to overall well-being.

Brief Overview of Natural Remedies

Natural remedies encompass a spectrum of holistic approaches to managing herpes that leverage lifestyle adjustments, dietary interventions, and herbal solutions. They play a complementary role alongside conventional treatments, aiming to reduce symptoms, support immune health, and enhance overall well-being.

Key Elements:

1. Lifestyle Adjustments: Emphasizing the importance of a balanced diet, hydration, and stress management for immune health.

2. Herbal Supplements: Harnessing the antiviral properties of herbs like Echinacea, Lemon Balm, and Licorice Root to mitigate symptoms and support the body's defense mechanisms.

3. Topical Applications: Utilizing natural elements such as Aloe Vera, Coconut Oil, and Tea Tree Oil for soothing relief on skin lesions.

Importance:
-Complementary Approach: Natural remedies work synergistically with conventional treatments to provide a comprehensive strategy for herpes management.

- Holistic Wellness: They contribute to overall well-being by addressing not only the symptoms but also factors influencing immune health and emotional balance.

Examples:
- Echinacea: Known for its immune-boosting properties.

- Aloe Vera: Offers soothing effects when applied topically to affected areas.

- Probiotics: Support gut health, influencing the body's immune response.

As we delve deeper into each element, this chapter aims to empower individuals with practical insights, fostering a balanced and integrative approach to herpes management.

Complementary Role Alongside Conventional Treatments

Natural remedies serve as valuable complements to conventional treatments for herpes, creating a harmonious synergy that addresses the virus on multiple fronts. While antiviral medications focus on directly combating the virus, natural remedies offer benefits such as immune system support, symptom alleviation, and overall well-being enhancement. Importantly, these natural approaches often come with minimal side effects compared to pharmaceutical interventions, contributing to a more favorable and holistic treatment experience.

The beauty of this complementary relationship lies in the holistic nature of natural remedies. They don't merely target symptoms but contribute to the body's resilience, fostering a robust immune response. Unlike some pharmaceuticals that may have side effects, natural remedies, when used judiciously, often exhibit a gentler profile. This combination allows individuals to benefit from the precision of conventional treatments and the nurturing qualities of natural approaches, offering a comprehensive strategy that aligns with the body's innate healing mechanisms.

Lifestyle and Dietary Considerations

Importance of a Balanced Diet

A balanced diet holds paramount importance in the treatment of herpes, playing a pivotal role in supporting the body's immune response and mitigating symptoms. Nutrient-rich foods, including fruits, vegetables, whole grains, and lean proteins, provide essential vitamins and minerals that fortify the immune system. Adequate hydration is equally crucial, aiding in overall health and assisting the body in flushing out toxins. A balanced diet helps maintain optimal body weight, reducing the risk of complications associated with herpes. Additionally, steering clear of processed foods and excessive arginine-rich foods can mitigate potential triggers for outbreaks. In essence, a balanced diet acts as a cornerstone, empowering individuals with the nutritional foundation needed to manage herpes effectively and enhance their overall well-being.

Nutrient-Rich Foods

Nutrient-Rich Foods for Herpes Treatment:

A robust and nutrient-rich diet plays a pivotal role in managing herpes by supporting the immune system and mitigating the frequency and intensity of outbreaks. Delving into specific nutrients and their food sources provides a comprehensive understanding of how dietary choices can impact herpes management.

1. Vitamin C:
   - Foods: Citrus fruits (oranges, grapefruits), strawberries, bell peppers.
   - Benefits: Vitamin C is renowned for its immune-boosting properties. It stimulates the production of

white blood cells, crucial defenders against infections. Additionally, it aids in collagen formation, contributing to the maintenance of healthy skin—a key aspect in managing herpes symptoms.

2. Vitamin E:
   - Foods: Almonds, sunflower seeds, spinach.
   - Benefits: Vitamin E functions as a potent antioxidant, neutralizing free radicals that may compromise the immune system. By bolstering immune response, it supports the body's ability to combat herpes outbreaks effectively.

3. Zinc:
   - Foods: Legumes (chickpeas, lentils), seeds, nuts.
   - Benefits: Zinc is indispensable for immune function and wound healing. It plays a crucial role in the replication of immune cells, helping the body mount a robust defense against the herpes virus. Additionally, zinc possesses anti-inflammatory properties, contributing to overall health.

 4. Lysine:
   -Foods: Lean proteins (chicken, turkey, fish), dairy, legumes.

- Benefits: Lysine is an amino acid that has been studied for its potential to inhibit the replication of the herpes simplex virus. It competes with arginine, another amino acid, limiting the availability of arginine for viral replication.

5. Omega-3 Fatty Acids:
   - Foods: Fatty fish (salmon, mackerel), chia seeds, walnuts.
   - Benefits: Omega-3 fatty acids are renowned for their anti-inflammatory effects. Chronic inflammation can exacerbate herpes symptoms, and incorporating omega-3-rich foods helps modulate the inflammatory response, contributing to overall well-being.

6. Quercetin:
   - Foods: Apples, onions, berries.
   - Benefits: Quercetin is a flavonoid with antiviral and anti-inflammatory properties. It may help inhibit the replication of the herpes virus and reduce inflammation, providing an additional layer of support in managing symptoms.

Incorporating these nutrient-rich foods into daily meals provides a foundation for a well-rounded diet that actively supports immune health and contributes to the effective management of herpes symptoms. The recipes not only deliver essential nutrients but also add a flavorful and diverse dimension to a herpes-friendly diet. As with any dietary adjustments, individual preferences and considerations should guide choices, and consulting with a healthcare professional or nutritionist is recommended to tailor these suggestions to personal needs and circumstances.

Sample recipes for Herpes treatment
1. Citrus Berry Smoothie:
   - Ingredients: Oranges, berries, yogurt, honey.
   - Preparation:
      - Squeeze fresh orange juice.
      - In a blender, combine the orange juice, a handful of berries, a scoop of yogurt, and a drizzle of honey.
      - Blend until smooth.
      - Pour into a glass and garnish with additional berries.

2. Spinach and Almond Salad:
   - Ingredients: Spinach, almonds, cherry tomatoes, feta cheese.
   - Preparation:
      - Wash and dry the spinach leaves.

- Toast almonds in a dry pan until lightly browned.
- In a bowl, combine spinach, halved cherry tomatoes, toasted almonds, and crumbled feta cheese.
- Toss the salad gently.
- Drizzle with olive oil and balsamic vinegar before serving.

3. Grilled Salmon with Quinoa:
  - Ingredients: Salmon, quinoa, lemon, herbs.
  - Preparation:
    - Season the salmon fillets with salt, pepper, and herbs of your choice.
    - Grill the salmon until cooked through.
    - Cook quinoa according to package instructions.
    - Serve the grilled salmon over a bed of cooked quinoa.
    - Squeeze fresh lemon juice over the dish before serving.

4. Chickpea and Spinach Curry:
  - Ingredients: Chickpeas, spinach, tomatoes, curry spices.
  - Preparation:
    - In a pot, sauté onions and garlic until softened.

- Add curry spices (turmeric, cumin, coriander) and stir.
- Pour in canned tomatoes and cooked chickpeas.
- Simmer until flavors meld.
- Add fresh spinach and cook until wilted.
- Serve over rice or with naan bread.

5. Berry-Infused Chia Pudding:
- Ingredients: Berries, chia seeds, almond milk, honey.
- Preparation:
- In a bowl, mix chia seeds with almond milk.
- Let it sit in the refrigerator for a few hours or overnight until it thickens.
- Layer the chia pudding with fresh berries in a glass or bowl.
- Drizzle honey on top for sweetness.
- Enjoy as a healthy dessert or breakfast.

These recipes not only provide essential nutrients for managing herpes but also introduce flavorful and satisfying options to your daily meals. Adjustments can be made based on personal preferences and dietary restrictions. Always consult with a healthcare professional or nutritionist for personalized advice tailored to individual needs.

Foods to Avoid or Limit

Avoiding or limiting certain foods can be beneficial in managing herpes outbreaks. While individual tolerance to specific foods may vary, here are general guidelines on foods to avoid or limit:

1. Arginine-Rich Foods:
   - Examples: Nuts (especially peanuts), seeds (like sunflower and pumpkin seeds), chocolate, and some grains.
   - Reason: Arginine promotes the replication of the herpes virus, potentially triggering outbreaks. Balancing arginine intake with lysine-rich foods is essential.

2. High-Arginine Proteins:
   - Examples: Red meat, particularly beef.
   - Reason: Red meat can be high in arginine, contributing to potential outbreak triggers. Consider leaner protein sources.

3. Processed Foods and Sugars:

- Examples: Sugary snacks, sodas, and processed foods.
- Reason: High sugar intake may compromise the immune system and exacerbate inflammation, potentially influencing the frequency and severity of outbreaks.

4. Alcohol:
- Reason: Alcohol can weaken the immune system and dehydrate the body, potentially impacting the ability to manage herpes symptoms effectively.

5. Acidic Foods:
- Examples: Citrus fruits, tomatoes, and vinegar.
- Reason: These foods may irritate oral herpes lesions, potentially worsening symptoms.

6. Excessive Caffeine:
- Reason: While moderate caffeine intake is generally acceptable, excessive caffeine can contribute to stress and impact sleep, factors that may influence herpes outbreaks.

7. Processed and Fried Foods:
- Examples: Fast food, fried snacks.

- Reason: These foods may contain high levels of unhealthy fats and lack essential nutrients, potentially affecting overall health and immune function.

8. Dairy Products High in L-Arginine:
   - Examples: Full-fat dairy products.
   - Reason: Some dairy products can be high in arginine, so choosing lower-arginine options may be beneficial.

Individual responses to these foods can vary, and it's essential to pay attention to personal triggers. Maintaining a balanced diet, rich in lysine-containing foods, and being mindful of potential trigger foods can contribute to a holistic approach in managing herpes. Consulting with a healthcare professional or nutritionist for personalized guidance is recommended.

Hydration and Its Impact on Immune Health

Proper hydration is a cornerstone of overall health, and its influence on immune function is profound. Adequate water intake is not only essential for physiological processes but also plays a crucial role in supporting a robust immune system. Here's an exploration of how hydration impacts immune health:

1. Cellular Function:
   - Water's Role: Water is a fundamental component of cells, facilitating various biochemical reactions crucial for immune cell function.
   - Impact: Well-hydrated cells function optimally, contributing to a more effective immune response.

2. Lymphatic System Support:
   - Lymphatic Fluid: The lymphatic system, a key part of the immune system, relies on adequate hydration. Lymph, a fluid within the lymphatic system, transports immune cells and removes waste products.
   - Impact: Proper hydration supports the flow of lymph, enhancing the transport of immune cells throughout the body.

3. Detoxification and Waste Removal:
   - Water's Role: Hydration aids in the elimination of toxins and waste products through urine.
   - Impact: Efficient removal of waste products ensures a cleaner internal environment, reducing the burden on the immune system.

4. Mucous Membrane Integrity:
   - Water Content:bMucous membranes, present in the respiratory and gastrointestinal tracts, require sufficient hydration to maintain their integrity.
   - Impact: Hydrated mucous membranes serve as a physical barrier, preventing pathogens from entering the body and initiating infections.

5. Temperature Regulation:
   - Water's Role: Sweat, produced during hydration, assists in temperature regulation.
   - Impact: Maintaining a stable body temperature supports overall immune function, as extreme temperatures can stress the body and compromise immune responses.

6. Prevention of Dehydration-Induced Stress:
   - Dehydration Stress: Dehydration can induce stress on the body, releasing stress hormones.
   - Impact: Prolonged stress can suppress immune function, making adequate hydration crucial for mitigating stress-related immune suppression.

Tips for Optimal Hydration:
1. Water Intake: Aim for at least 8 glasses (64 ounces) of water per day, adjusting based on

individual needs, climate, and physical activity levels.

2. Electrolyte Balance: Include foods rich in electrolytes, such as fruits and vegetables, to maintain a balance that supports proper cellular function.

3. Consistent Hydration: Drink water consistently throughout the day rather than consuming large amounts at once.

4. Monitor Urine Color: Pale yellow urine is a good indicator of adequate hydration, while dark yellow may signal dehydration.

5. Hydration with Herbal Teas: Unsweetened herbal teas can contribute to hydration while providing additional health benefits.

Understanding the integral role of hydration in immune health emphasizes the importance of maintaining a well-hydrated state for overall well-being and effective immune responses.

Stress Management Techniques

Impact of stress on herpes

Stress can exert a significant impact on the course of herpes infections, particularly those caused by the herpes simplex virus (HSV-1 and HSV-2). The relationship between stress and herpes is complex, involving intricate interactions between the immune system, neural pathways, and the reactivation of the virus. Here's a detailed exploration of how stress influences herpes:

1. Stress Hormones and Immune Response:
   - Cortisol Release: Stress triggers the release of cortisol, a stress hormone.
   - Immune Suppression: Prolonged exposure to elevated cortisol levels can suppress the immune system, potentially diminishing its ability to control herpes outbreaks.

2. Herpes Reactivation:
   - Neuroendocrine Connection: The nervous and endocrine systems are intricately linked. Stress signals may influence the nervous system,

potentially leading to the reactivation of latent herpes viruses.

- Viral Shedding: Reactivation can result in viral shedding, increasing the risk of transmission to others.

3. Increased Frequency and Severity of Outbreaks:

- Association with Stress: Research suggests a correlation between high-stress levels and an increased frequency and severity of herpes outbreaks.

- Individual Variability: Responses to stress vary, and not everyone with herpes experiences outbreaks in direct correlation with stress. However, stress remains a recognized trigger for many individuals.

4. Impact on Immune Modulation:

- Chronic Stress: Chronic stress may lead to dysregulation of the immune system, affecting its ability to maintain herpes in a dormant state.

- Inflammation: Stress-induced inflammation can create an environment conducive to viral replication.

5. Emotional Well-being and Coping Mechanisms:

- Psychological Impact: Living with herpes can induce emotional stress, creating a feedback loop that may exacerbate physical symptoms.
   - Coping Strategies: Effective stress management and coping strategies are crucial for minimizing the impact of emotional stress on herpes.

Stress Management Strategies for Herpes

1. Mindfulness and Relaxation Techniques'
   - Meditation, deep breathing exercises, and mindfulness practices can help reduce stress levels.

2. Regular Exercise:
   - Physical activity is known to alleviate stress and positively impact immune function.

3. Social Support:
   - Seeking support from friends, family, or support groups can provide emotional assistance in coping with the emotional aspects of herpes.

4. Counseling or Therapy:
   - Professional counseling can offer a structured approach to managing stress and emotional challenges.

5. Balanced Lifestyle:
  - Aim for a balanced lifestyle with adequate sleep, a healthy diet, and regular physical activity.

6. Physical Activity: Regular physical activity is a potent stress reduction technique. Exercise releases endorphins, the body's natural mood enhancers, promoting a sense of well-being and mitigating the impact of stress on mental health.

Understanding and managing stress are integral components of herpes care. By adopting effective stress management strategies, individuals can potentially reduce the frequency and severity of outbreaks and support overall well-being in the context of herpes infections. Always consult with healthcare professionals for personalized guidance based on individual circumstances.

Chapter 4

Herbal Supplements and Extracts

Embark on a journey into the healing power of nature. Chapter 4 delves into herbal supplements and extracts, unlocking their potential to complement herpes management. Explore nature's pharmacy and discover pathways to symptom relief, immune support, and holistic well-being.

Echinacea

Echinacea, a flowering plant native to North America, is renowned for its immune-boosting properties. Packed with bioactive compounds, it stimulates immune cells to enhance the body's natural defenses. Whether in herbal teas or supplements, Echinacea stands as a potent ally in fortifying the immune system against infections.

Lemon Balm (Melissa officinalis)
While lemon balm (Melissa officinalis) has been studied for its potential antiviral properties, research on its effectiveness specifically against herpes simplex virus (HSV) is limited and inconclusive. Some studies suggest it may have antiviral effects, but more research is needed to establish its efficacy and safety for treating HSV. It's essential to consult with a healthcare professional before using herbal remedies for medical conditions.

Licorice Root

Licorice root has been investigated for its potential antiviral properties, including activity against herpes simplex virus (HSV). Glycyrrhizin, a compound found in licorice root, has demonstrated antiviral effects in some studies. However, it's important to note that the evidence is not conclusive, and more research is needed to determine the effectiveness of licorice root specifically for treating HSV.

Additionally, prolonged or excessive consumption of licorice root can have side effects, such as elevated blood pressure and potassium imbalance. It's crucial to consult with a healthcare professional before using licorice root or any herbal remedy, especially for managing medical conditions like HSV.

Topical Remedies

Aloe Vera Gel

Aloe vera, derived from the succulent plant's leaves, has gained popularity for its potential medicinal properties. While some people use aloe vera gel to alleviate discomfort associated with skin conditions, it's important to note that there is limited scientific evidence supporting its efficacy as a specific treatment for HSV lesions.

Aloe vera is known for its soothing and moisturizing effects, which may provide temporary relief from itching or irritation. The gel contains various bioactive compounds, including polysaccharides, anthraquinones, and phytosterols, contributing to its anti-inflammatory and antimicrobial properties. However, these properties do not necessarily guarantee a direct impact on HSV.

Research on aloe vera and HSV is relatively sparse, and the existing studies may not offer conclusive evidence. Herpes simplex virus infections, whether oral (HSV-1) or genital (HSV-2), typically require antiviral medications prescribed by healthcare professionals for effective management. These medications aim to control viral replication and reduce the frequency and severity of outbreaks.

While aloe vera may provide some comfort for individuals experiencing HSV-related skin discomfort, it is not a substitute for medically prescribed antiviral treatments. It's crucial to consult with a healthcare professional for appropriate guidance on managing HSV symptoms and outbreaks.

Moreover, individual responses to topical treatments can vary, and what works for one person may not be equally effective for another. Always prioritize open communication with healthcare providers to ensure the most suitable and evidence-based approach to managing herpes simplex virus infections.

Coconut Oil

Coconut oil has gained attention for its potential health benefits, and some individuals explore its use as a topical treatment for conditions like herpes simplex virus (HSV) lesions. Coconut oil is rich in fatty acids, particularly lauric acid, which exhibits antimicrobial properties. Here's a more in-depth look at the potential considerations:

1. Antimicrobial Properties: Lauric acid, a major component of coconut oil, has been studied for its antimicrobial effects. It may exert antiviral activity by disrupting lipid membranes of viruses, potentially inhibiting the replication of certain viruses, including

HSV. However, the evidence supporting coconut oil as a definitive treatment for HSV is limited.

2. Anti-Inflammatory Effects: Coconut oil contains compounds with anti-inflammatory properties, which might help alleviate some of the discomfort associated with HSV lesions. Reducing inflammation can contribute to symptom relief.

3. Moisturizing Properties: The emollient nature of coconut oil can provide moisture to the skin, potentially preventing dryness and promoting overall skin health. This moisturizing effect may be beneficial for individuals experiencing skin irritation due to HSV.

4. Individual Responses: Responses to topical treatments can vary among individuals. While some may find relief from using coconut oil, it's essential to recognize that its effectiveness might differ from person to person.

5. Cautionary Notes: Although coconut oil is generally considered safe for external use, it may not be suitable for everyone. Individuals with coconut allergies should avoid using coconut oil. Additionally, as with any alternative treatment, it is

crucial to consult with a healthcare professional before relying solely on coconut oil for managing HSV.

6. Complementary Approach: Coconut oil should be seen as a complementary or supportive measure rather than a primary or standalone treatment for HSV. Medically prescribed antiviral medications remain the primary approach for managing herpes simplex virus infections.

Safe Application Guidelines

When considering the topical application of coconut oil for conditions like herpes simplex virus (HSV) lesions, it's important to follow safe application guidelines:

1. Cleanliness: Wash the affected area with mild soap and water before applying coconut oil. Keeping the area clean helps prevent infection and promotes effective absorption of the oil.

2. Quality of Coconut Oil: Choose a high-quality, organic, and cold-pressed coconut oil. This ensures that you are using a pure form without added chemicals or preservatives.

3. Patch Test: Before widespread application, perform a patch test by applying a small amount of coconut oil to a small area of skin. Monitor for any adverse reactions, such as redness or irritation. If irritation occurs, discontinue use.

4. Gentle Application: Apply coconut oil gently to the affected area using clean hands or a cotton swab. Avoid rubbing vigorously, especially if the lesions are tender.

5. Frequency: Apply coconut oil as needed, but avoid excessive application. Overapplication may not necessarily increase effectiveness and could lead to unnecessary irritation.

6. Hygiene Practices: To prevent the spread of the virus, avoid using your fingers to apply coconut oil directly. Instead, use a disposable applicator or wash your hands thoroughly before and after application.

7. Combination with Medications: If you are already using prescribed antiviral medications, continue following your healthcare provider's instructions.

Coconut oil can be a complementary measure, but it should not replace prescribed medications.

8. Individual Sensitivity: Be mindful of individual sensitivities. If you experience any worsening of symptoms or new reactions after applying coconut oil, consult with a healthcare professional.

9. Avoid Eye Contact: Be cautious to avoid getting coconut oil in the eyes. If accidental contact occurs, rinse thoroughly with water.

10. Consult a Healthcare Professional: Before incorporating coconut oil or any alternative treatment, consult with a healthcare professional. They can provide personalized advice based on your specific health condition and medical history.

Remember that while coconut oil may offer some relief for skin conditions, it is not a substitute for professional medical advice and prescribed treatments. If you have concerns about managing herpes simplex virus infections, seek guidance from a healthcare provider.

Tea Tree Oil

Tea tree oil, derived from the leaves of the Melaleuca alternifolia tree, is known for its antimicrobial and anti-inflammatory properties. Some individuals explore its use as a topical treatment for conditions like herpes simplex virus (HSV) lesions. Here are important considerations for safe application:

1. Dilution: Tea tree oil is potent and should be diluted before application to avoid skin irritation. Mix a few drops of tea tree oil with a carrier oil, such as coconut oil or jojoba oil, before applying to the affected area.

2. Patch Test: Before widespread use, perform a patch test by applying the diluted tea tree oil to a small area of skin. Monitor for any adverse reactions, and if irritation occurs, discontinue use.

3. Cleanliness: Clean the affected area with mild soap and water before applying diluted tea tree oil. This helps prevent infection and ensures proper absorption.

4. Gentle Application: Apply the diluted tea tree oil gently to the affected area using a clean cotton

swab or ball. Avoid excessive rubbing, especially if the lesions are tender.

5. Avoid Eye Contact: Be cautious not to get tea tree oil in the eyes. If accidental contact occurs, rinse thoroughly with water.

6. Frequency: Apply the diluted tea tree oil as needed, but avoid overuse. Using it excessively may not necessarily enhance its effectiveness and could lead to irritation.

7. Hygiene Practices: To prevent the spread of the virus, avoid using your fingers directly. Instead, use a disposable applicator or wash your hands thoroughly before and after application.

8. Combination with Medications: If you are already using prescribed antiviral medications, continue following your healthcare provider's instructions. Tea tree oil can be considered a complementary measure but should not replace prescribed medications.

9. Individual Sensitivity: Monitor for individual sensitivities. If you experience worsening symptoms

or new reactions after applying tea tree oil, consult with a healthcare professional.

10. Consult a Healthcare Professional: Before using tea tree oil or any alternative treatment, consult with a healthcare professional. They can provide personalized advice based on your specific health condition and medical history.

While tea tree oil may have potential benefits, it's important to approach its use cautiously and as a complementary measure rather than a primary treatment for HSV. Always seek guidance from a healthcare provider for the most appropriate and evidence-based approach to managing herpes simplex virus infections.

Dilution and Application Instructions

Here are general dilution and application instructions for using tea tree oil as a topical treatment for conditions like herpes simplex virus (HSV) lesions:

Dilution:

1. Carrier Oil: Choose a suitable carrier oil such as coconut oil, jojoba oil, or almond oil.

2. Ratio: Mix a few drops of tea tree oil with a larger amount of the carrier oil. A common ratio is 1-2 drops of tea tree oil per teaspoon of carrier oil, but individual sensitivities may vary.

3. Patch Test: Before widespread use, perform a patch test by applying the diluted mixture to a small area of skin. Wait 24 hours and check for any adverse reactions, such as redness or irritation. If irritation occurs, discontinue use.

Application:

1. Clean the Area: Wash the affected area with mild soap and water. Pat the area dry gently.

2. Clean Hands: Ensure that your hands are clean before handling the diluted tea tree oil.

3. Use an Applicator: To avoid direct contact, use a clean cotton swab or ball to apply the diluted mixture to the affected area. Alternatively, disposable applicators can be used.

4. Gentle Application: Apply the diluted mixture gently to the affected area. Avoid vigorous rubbing, especially if the lesions are tender.

5. Avoid Eye Contact: Be cautious not to get the diluted mixture in the eyes. If accidental contact occurs, rinse thoroughly with water.

6. Frequency: Apply the diluted mixture as needed, but avoid overuse. Using it excessively may not necessarily enhance its effectiveness and could lead to irritation.

7. Hygiene Practices: To prevent the spread of the virus, avoid using your fingers directly. Wash your hands thoroughly before and after application.

8. Combination with Medications: If you are already using prescribed antiviral medications, continue following your healthcare provider's instructions. Tea tree oil can be considered a complementary measure but should not replace prescribed medications.

9. Monitor for Sensitivities: Pay attention to individual sensitivities. If you experience worsening

symptoms or new reactions after applying tea tree oil, consult with a healthcare professional.

10. Consult a Healthcare Professional: Before using tea tree oil or any alternative treatment, consult with a healthcare professional. They can provide personalized advice based on your specific health condition and medical history.

Always prioritize safety, and if you have concerns about managing herpes simplex virus infections, seek guidance from a healthcare provider.

Chapter 5

Probiotics and Immune Support

Role of Probiotics in Gut Health

Probiotics are live microorganisms, primarily bacteria and yeast, that confer health benefits when consumed in adequate amounts. Found in certain foods and supplements, they promote a balanced and healthy gut microbiota, supporting various aspects of digestion and immune function.

The role of probiotics in gut health, particularly in the context of herpes simplex virus (HSV) treatment, is an area of ongoing research. Probiotics are beneficial microorganisms, usually bacteria, that can confer health benefits when consumed in adequate amounts. Here are some considerations regarding the potential role of probiotics in managing HSV and supporting overall gut health:

1. Immune System Support: Probiotics may influence the immune system, and a healthy immune response is crucial for managing viral infections, including HSV. Some studies suggest that probiotics can modulate immune function and enhance the body's defense mechanisms.

2. Microbial Balance: Maintaining a balanced microbial environment in the gut is important for overall health. Probiotics contribute to this balance by promoting the growth of beneficial bacteria and inhibiting the overgrowth of harmful microorganisms. A balanced gut microbiota can positively influence the immune system's ability to respond to infections.

3. Anti-Inflammatory Effects: Chronic inflammation is associated with various health conditions, including viral infections. Probiotics may help reduce inflammation in the gut, which can indirectly support the body's ability to manage viral infections.

4. Gut-Brain Axis: There is a growing understanding of the gut-brain axis, which highlights the

bidirectional communication between the gut and the central nervous system. Probiotics may influence this communication, and a healthy gut environment could potentially contribute to overall well-being, including the management of stress, which is known to impact HSV outbreaks.

5. Antiviral Properties: Some research suggests that certain probiotic strains may have direct antiviral properties. However, more studies are needed to establish specific strains and their efficacy against HSV.

If you are considering incorporating probiotics into your routine, it's advisable to consult with a healthcare professional. They can provide personalized advice based on your health status and help determine the most appropriate approach to support gut health in the context of managing HSV or other health conditions.

Probiotic-Rich Foods

Probiotic-rich foods contain live beneficial microorganisms that contribute to a healthy gut microbiota. Some examples of probiotic-rich foods include:

1. Yogurt: Choose plain, unsweetened yogurt with live cultures. Greek yogurt and traditional yogurt are good options.

2. Kefir: A fermented dairy product that resembles a drinkable yogurt, kefir is rich in probiotics.

3. Sauerkraut: Fermented cabbage that provides a source of beneficial bacteria. Choose unpasteurized sauerkraut for live cultures.

4. Kimchi: A traditional Korean dish made from fermented vegetables, usually cabbage and radishes, seasoned with spices.

5. Miso: A Japanese seasoning produced by fermenting soybeans with salt and koji (a type of fungus). It is commonly used in soups.

6. Tempeh: Fermented soybean product with a firm texture and nutty flavor. It is a popular meat substitute.

7. Pickles (in brine): Pickled cucumbers fermented in a saltwater solution, not in vinegar, to retain live cultures.

8. Traditional Buttermilk: The liquid left behind after churning butter from fermented cream. It differs from cultured buttermilk found in some stores.

9. Natto: A traditional Japanese dish made from fermented soybeans. It has a distinctive texture and flavor.

10. Lassi: A traditional Indian drink made with yogurt, water, and spices, often flavored with fruits or herbs.

Incorporating a variety of probiotic-rich foods into your diet can contribute to a diverse and balanced gut microbiota, supporting overall digestive and immune health. Always choose options with live cultures and, if possible, avoid excessive processing or heat treatment, as it may reduce the viability of probiotics.

Chapter 6

Integration into Daily Routine

Creating a Holistic Wellness Plan

Creating a holistic wellness plan involves addressing various aspects of your well-being, including physical, mental, emotional, and social aspects. Here's a simple guide to help you develop a holistic wellness plan:

1. **Assessment:**
   - Physical Health: Evaluate your current physical health, including exercise habits, nutrition, and sleep.
   - Mental and Emotional Well-being: Reflect on your stress levels, emotional balance, and mental health.

-Social Connections Consider the quality of your relationships and social support.

2. Set Clear Goals:
- Establish specific, measurable, achievable, relevant, and time-bound (SMART) goals for each aspect of well-being.
- Example: "Engage in 30 minutes of moderate exercise five times a week" or "Practice mindfulness for 10 minutes daily."

3. Physical Health:
- Exercise: Include a mix of aerobic, strength training, and flexibility exercises.
- Nutrition: Focus on a balanced and nutritious diet with a variety of fruits, vegetables, whole grains, and lean proteins.
- Sleep: Aim for 7-9 hours of quality sleep per night.

4. Mental and Emotional Well-being:
- Mindfulness and Relaxation Techniques: Incorporate practices like meditation, deep breathing, or yoga to manage stress.
- Therapeutic Activities: Consider counseling, therapy, or engaging in activities you enjoy to support mental well-being.

5. Social Connections:

- Build and Strengthen Relationships: Foster meaningful connections with family, friends, and community.
- Communication: Practice effective communication and express your needs to maintain healthy relationships.

6. Healthy Habits:

- Hydration: Ensure adequate water intake throughout the day.
- Limit Stimulants and Substances: Moderation in the consumption of caffeine, alcohol, and other substances.

7. Holistic Approaches:

- Probiotics and Nutrition: Include probiotic-rich foods for gut health, and prioritize nutrient-dense foods.
- Nature and Outdoor Time: Spend time in nature for relaxation and stress reduction.
- Holistic Therapies: Explore complementary therapies like acupuncture, massage, or herbal remedies with the guidance of healthcare professionals.

8. Regular Check-ins:

   - Periodically reassess your goals and adjust your wellness plan as needed.
   - Celebrate achievements and recognize areas for improvement.

9. Professional Guidance:

   - Consult with healthcare professionals, nutritionists, or mental health professionals as needed.
   - Consider holistic healthcare providers who approach well-being from a comprehensive perspective.

10. Consistency and Self-Compassion:

   - Strive for consistency rather than perfection.
   - Be kind to yourself and recognize that well-being is an ongoing journey.

Remember that a holistic wellness plan is unique to each individual, so tailor it to your preferences, values, and health needs. Regularly revisiting and adapting your plan will contribute to sustained well-being over time.

Tracking and Evaluating Progress

Here are five key steps for tracking and evaluating progress in your holistic wellness plan:

1. Regular Self-Reflection:
   - Take time to reflect on your overall well-being regularly.
   - Assess how you feel physically, mentally, and emotionally.
   - Consider any changes in your habits and behaviors.

2. Quantifiable Metrics:
   - Set specific, measurable goals for different aspects of your wellness.
   - Track quantifiable metrics such as exercise frequency, sleep duration, or stress levels.
   - Use wellness apps or journals to record and monitor progress.

3. Objective Measurements:
   - Establish baseline measurements for physical health, like weight or blood pressure.
   - Periodically reassess these measurements to gauge changes over time.
   - Adjust goals based on objective data.

4. Celebrate Achievements:
  - Recognize and celebrate your accomplishments, both big and small.
  - Positive reinforcement can motivate continued effort and commitment.

5. Feedback and Professional Guidance:
  - Seek feedback from friends, family, or healthcare professionals.
  - External perspectives can provide insights and encouragement.
  - Regularly consult with professionals for assessments and adjustments to your wellness plan.

Consistent application of these steps will contribute to effective tracking, evaluation, and refinement of your holistic wellness plan.

Long-Term Maintenance Strategies

When it comes to long-term maintenance of herpes treatment, consider the following strategies:

1. Medication Adherence: Follow your healthcare provider's prescribed antiviral medications consistently to manage and reduce outbreaks.

2. Regular Medical Check-ups: Schedule regular follow-up appointments with your healthcare provider to monitor your condition, discuss any concerns, and adjust treatment if necessary.

3. Healthy Lifestyle: Maintain a healthy lifestyle with a balanced diet, regular exercise, and sufficient sleep. These factors can positively impact your immune system.

4. Stress Management: Since stress can trigger herpes outbreaks, incorporate stress-reduction techniques such as meditation, yoga, or counseling into your routine.

5. Avoid Triggers: Identify and avoid factors that may trigger outbreaks, such as certain foods, excessive sunlight exposure, or other environmental factors.

6. Safe Practices: If sexually active, communicate openly with your partner, practice safe sex, and use protection to reduce the risk of transmission.

7. Educate Yourself: Stay informed about herpes, its symptoms, and any new developments in treatments. This knowledge empowers you to make informed decisions about your health.

Always consult with your healthcare provider for personalized advice and adjustments to your treatment plan based on your specific needs and circumstances.

Chapter 7

Prevention and Risk Reduction

Safe Practices and Vaccination

To help prevent HSV (Herpes Simplex Virus) transmission:

1. Safe Practices:
   - Use condoms consistently and correctly during sexual activity.
   - Limit sexual partners and choose partners who have been tested and are HSV-free.
   - Avoid sexual contact during outbreaks or if symptoms are present.

2. Regular Health Check-ups:
   - Attend regular check-ups with a healthcare professional to discuss sexual health and screenings.

3. Open Communication:

- Communicate openly with your partner about sexual health, history, and any concerns.

Emotional and Psychological Support

Navigating the Emotional Impact

Coping with the emotional impact of having HSV (Herpes Simplex Virus) can be challenging, but there are ways to navigate it:

1. Education:
   - Learn about HSV to dispel myths and reduce anxiety. Understanding the virus can empower you to make informed decisions.

2. Open Communication:
   - Talk to your partner about your diagnosis. Open communication fosters understanding and support.

3. Support Groups:
   - Join HSV support groups or seek counseling to connect with others who share similar experiences.

4. Professional Guidance:

- Consult with healthcare professionals or therapists to address emotional concerns and receive guidance on managing the psychological impact.

5. Self-Compassion:
   - Be kind to yourself. Remember that having HSV does not define your worth or identity.

6. Disclosure:
   - When ready, disclose your status to potential partners. Honesty can build trust and alleviate anxiety.

7. Maintain Healthy Relationships:
   - Surround yourself with supportive friends and family who understand and respect your journey.

8. Focus on Overall Well-Being:
   - Prioritize self-care, including proper nutrition, exercise, and sufficient sleep to support your physical and mental health.

Remember, you are not alone, and seeking emotional support is a crucial part of navigating the challenges associated with HSV.

Strategies for Coping and Resilience

1. Deep Breathing:
   - Practice deep, slow breaths to calm your nervous system and reduce stress.

2. Gratitude Journal:
   - Regularly jot down things you're grateful for to shift focus towards positive aspects of life.

3. Connect with Nature:
   - Spend time outdoors. Nature has a calming effect and can help alleviate stress.

4. Stay Present:
   - Focus on the current moment rather than worrying about the past or future. Mindfulness can enhance resilience.

5. Exercise Regularly:
   - Engage in physical activity to release endorphins and boost your mood, contributing to overall resilience.

Dispelling Myths and Reducing Stigma

Let's address some common myths about HSV (Herpes Simplex Virus) to dispel misinformation:

1. Myth: HSV Only Affects Promiscuous Individuals.
   - Fact: HSV can be transmitted through various forms of sexual contact, and anyone, regardless of sexual activity, can contract the virus.

2. Myth: HSV Always Causes Visible Symptoms.
   - Fact: Many individuals with HSV may not exhibit noticeable symptoms. Asymptomatic carriers can still transmit the virus to others.

3. Myth: HSV is Always Sexually Transmitted.
   - Fact: While sexual contact is a common mode of transmission, HSV can also be transmitted through non-sexual contact, such as kissing or touching.

4. Myth: HSV is a Rare Condition.
   - Fact: HSV is widespread. The World Health Organization (WHO) estimates that over 3.7 billion people under the age of 50 have HSV-1, and around 491 million people aged 15-49 have HSV-2 globally.

5. Myth: You Can Only Get HSV Once.

  - Fact: HSV is a lifelong infection, and while outbreaks may decrease over time, the virus remains in the body. Reinfection with a different strain is also possible.

It's crucial to base our understanding of HSV on accurate information to reduce stigma and promote a more informed and compassionate perspective.

www.ingramcontent.com/pod-product-compliance
Lightning Source LLC
Chambersburg PA
CBHW071054260726
48661CB00006B/2272